KETO ICE CREAM

Discover 30 Easy to Follow Ketogenic Cookbook Ice Cream recipes for Your Low-Carb Diet with Gluten-Free and wheat to Maximize your weight loss

STEPHANIE BAKER

Copyright © Stephanie Baker

All rights reserved. No part of this book may be reproduced, scanned or distributed in any printed or electronic form without permission. Please do not participate in or encourage piracy of copyrighted materials in violation of the author's rights. Purchase only authorized editions.

1
LOW CARB CINNAMON ICE CREAM

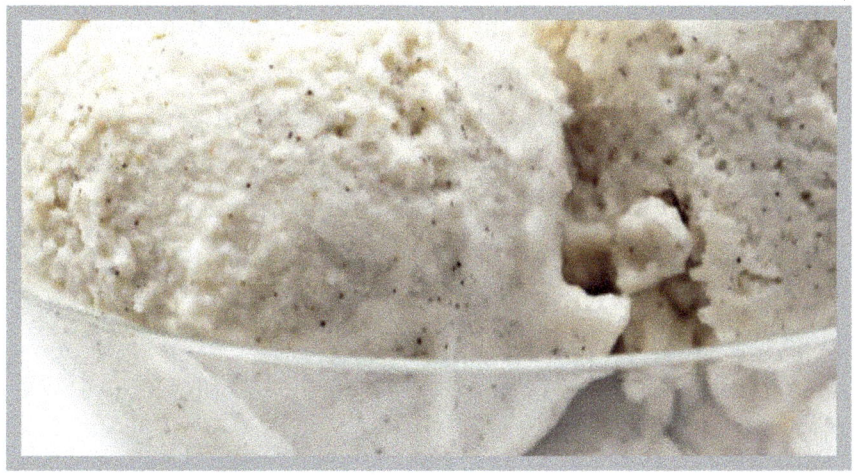

5 minutes.

INGREDIENTS

. . .

50 G OF POWDERED ERYTHRITOL *

    40 g of xylitol * ground into powder

    1 g of xanthan gum * or guar or 1.5 g of locust bean gum

    150ml vegan coconut milk, alternatively milk (3.5%)

    70 g cream n.B. vegan

    1 inulin * or vodka

    2 teaspoons of Ceylon cinnamon *

PREPARATION

Preparation with the ice cream maker

Mix erythritol, xylitol, xanthan, inulin and cinnamon.

Add the coconut milk and cream and mix everything until smooth.

Pour the mixture into the refrigerator and let it freeze.

Preparation without machine for ice cream

Mix erythritol, xylitol, xanthan, inulin and cinnamon.

Add the coconut milk and mix everything until smooth.

Whip the cream until compact and incorporate it.

Freeze the ice cream mass and, if possible, stir every 30-60 minutes so that as few ice crystals as possible are formed.

NUTRITIONAL VALUES

Serving size: 100 g | Calories: 126 kcal | Carbohydrates: 2.8 g | Protein: 1.9 g | Fat: 8.4 g

② SUGAR FREE RICE PUDDING ICE CREAM

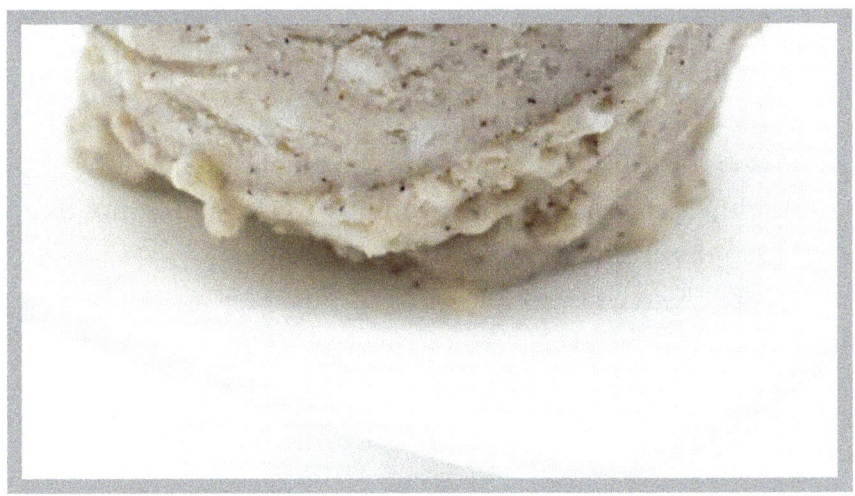

10 MIN.

INGREDIENTS

. . .

150 G OF COTTAGE cheese
70 ml of cream n.B. vegan
50 g of powdered erythritol *
40 g of xylitol * ground into powder
1 g of xanthan gum * or guar or 1.5 g of locust bean gum
1 inulin * or vodka
1 teaspoon of Ceylon cinnamon *

PREPARATION

Preparation with the ice cream maker
Mix erythritol, xylitol, xanthan, cinnamon and inulin.
Add ricotta and cream and mix everything until smooth.
Pour the mixture into the refrigerator and let it freeze.
Preparation without machine for ice cream
Mix erythritol, xylitol, xanthan, cinnamon and inulin.
Add the ricotta and mix everything together until smooth.
Whip the cream until thick and incorporate it.
Freeze the ice cream mass and, if possible, stir every 30-60 minutes so that as few ice crystals as possible are formed.

③
STRACCIATELLA ICE CREAM WITHOUT SUGAR

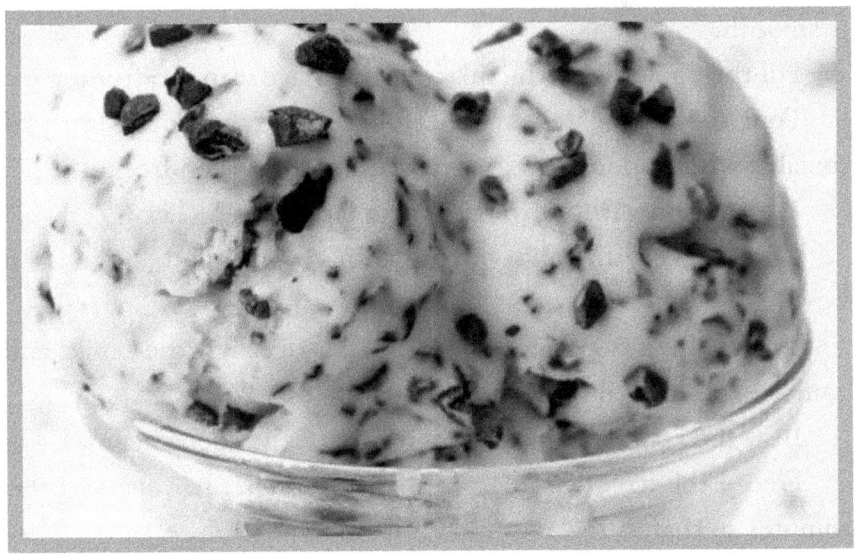

10 MINUTES.

INGREDIENTS

150 ml of milk (3.5%) or coconut milk (vegan version)
70 g of cream n.B. vegan
50 g of erythritol powder *
40 g xylitol * ground into powder
30 g cocoa beans *
1 tablespoon inulin * or vodka
1 g xanthan gum * or guar gum or 1.5 g locust bean gum
Vanilla extract * to taste

PREPARATION

Preparation with the ice cream machine

Mix erythritol, xylitol, xanthan, and inulin.

Stir in the milk, cream, and vanilla extract until the mixture is smooth.

Fill the cooler with the mixture and place it in the freezer.

Pour the ice into a freezer-safe jar until it is frozen but still mixable with a spoon. Mix in the cocoa beans, then freeze.

Preparation without the use of an ice cream maker

Combine erythritol, xylitol, xanthan gum, and inulin in a bowl.

TAKE In a separate bowl, whisk together the milk and vanilla extract until smooth.

Beat the cream until stiff and mix with the cocoa beans.

Freeze the ice cream batter and, if possible, stir every 30-60 minutes so that as few ice crystals form as possible.

4
MAKE YOURSELF SUGAR-FREE HAZELNUT ICE CREAM

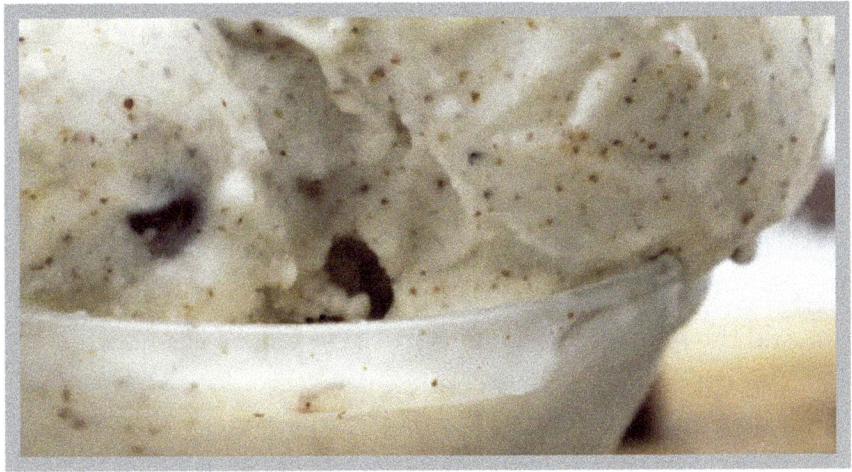

10 MINUTES.

INGREDIENTS
150 ml of milk (3.5%) or coconut milk (vegan version)

70 g of cream n.B. vegan

50 g hazelnut butter

50 g of erythritol powder *

40 g xylitol * ground into powder

30 g of chopped hazelnuts

1 g xanthan gum * or guar gum * or 1.5 g locust bean gum *

1 tablespoon inulin * or vodka

PREPARATION

Recipe for the refrigerator:

Mix erythritol, xylitol, xanthan, and inulin.

Add the milk, cream, and hazelnut butter and stir until smooth.

Pour the mixture into the cooler and let it freeze.

Finally, work the chopped hazelnuts.

Recipe without ice cream machine:

Mix erythritol, xylitol, xanthan gum, inulin, and chopped hazelnuts.

Add the milk and hazelnut butter and mix until smooth.

Beat the cream until stiff and work.

Freeze the ice cream batter and, if possible, stir every 30-60 minutes so that as few ice crystals form as possible.

6
LOW CARB SUGAR FREE VANILLA ICE CREAM

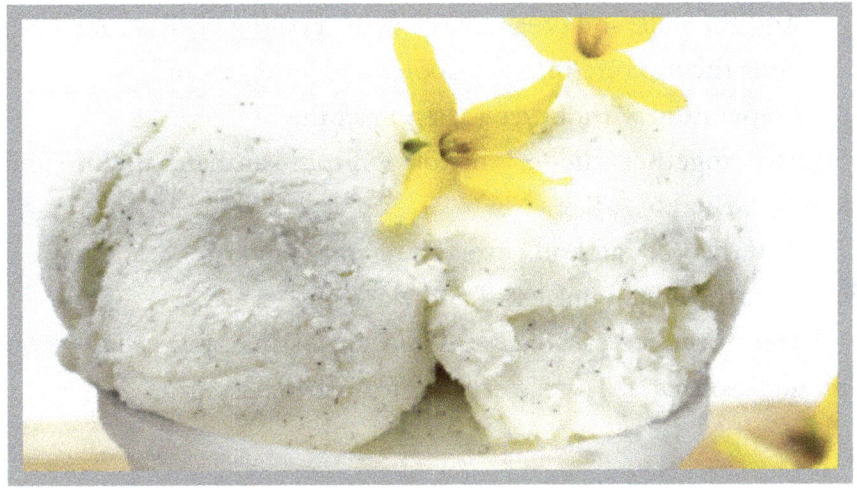

10 MINUTES.

INGREDIENTS
50 g of erythritol powder *

40 g xylitol * ground into powder
1 g xanthan gum * or guar gum * or 1.5 g locust bean gum *
150 ml of 3.5% milk or coconut milk (vegan version)
70 g of cream n.B. vegan
1 tablespoon inulin * or vodka
1 vanilla bean

PREPARATION

PREPARATION with the ice cream machine

Mix together the erythritol, xylitol, xanthan, inulin, and vanilla bean.

Add the milk and cream and mix everything until smooth.

Pour the mixture into the cooler and let it freeze.

Preparation without ice cream machine

Mix together the erythritol, xylitol, xanthan, inulin, and vanilla bean.

Add the milk and mix everything until smooth.

Beat the cream until stiff and work.

Freeze the ice cream batter and, if possible, stir every 30-60 minutes so that as few ice crystals form as possible.

7

GOLDEN ICE CREAM WITH TURMERIC, GINGER AND CINNAMON

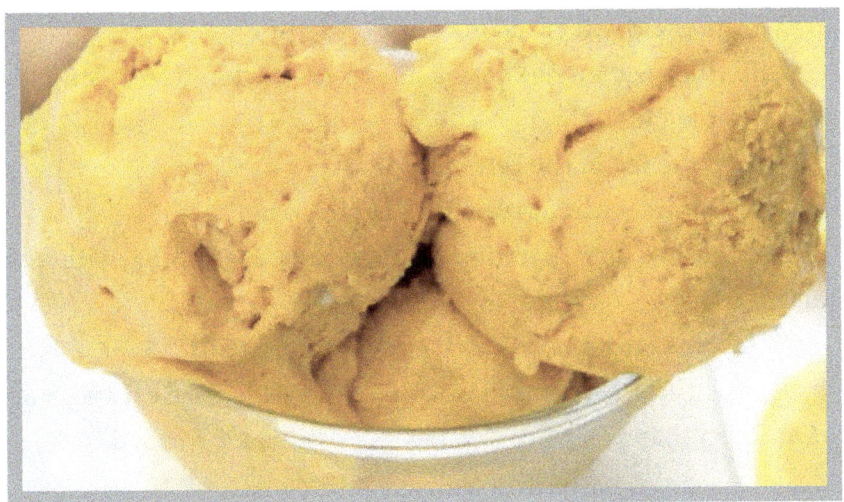

10 MIN.

INGREDIENTS

50 g of powdered erythritol *

40 g of xylitol * ground into powder

1 g of xanthan gum * or guar or 1.5 g of locust bean gum

150ml 3.5% milk or coconut milk (vegan version)

70 g cream n.B. vegan

1 inulin * or vodka

1 turmeric *

1/2 tablespoon of Ceylon cinnamon *

1 teaspoon finely grated fresh ginger

PREPARATION

Preparation with the ice cream maker

Mix all the dry ingredients.

USE the wet ingredients and mix everything until smooth with a stir stick.

Freeze the ice in the refrigerator.

Preparation without machine for ice cream

Mix all the dry ingredients, then mix everything with the milk.

Whip the cream until thick and incorporate it.

Freeze the ice cream mass and, if possible, stir every 30-60 minutes so that as few ice crystals as possible are formed.

8

GINGER WATER ICE CREAM WITH TURMERIC

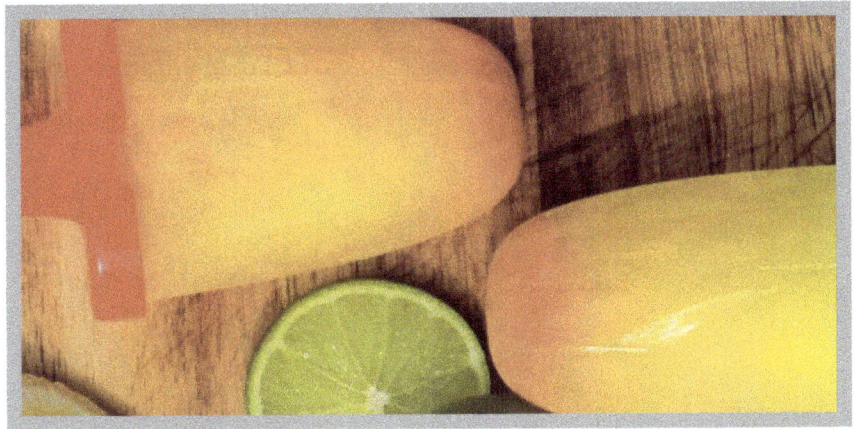

10 MIN.

INGREDIENTS

- 1 liter of water
- 1 piece of ginger approx. 5 cm

1 teaspoon of turmeric *
1 organic lemon

PREPARATION

SCRAPE off the ginger and cut it into small pieces.

Rub the lemon peel and squeeze the juice.

Bring the water to a boil in a saucepan, add the ginger, turmeric and lemon peel and simmer for about 15 minutes.

Pour the ginger water through a sieve and let it cool to room temperature.

Add the lemon juice, pour it into the popsicles and freeze.
NUTRITIONAL VALUES

Serving size: 100 g | Calories: 0.4 kcal | Carbohydrates: 0.1 g

9

SUGAR FREE ICE CREAM CAKE

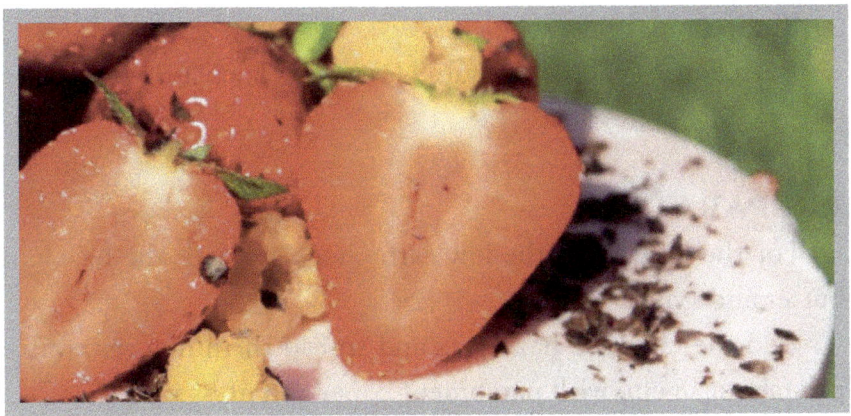

30 MINUTES.

INGREDIENTS

On the ground

85g chocolate or low-carb chocolate (at least 85% cocoa content), nB vegan

85 g of hazelnut butter

70 g of chopped hazelnuts

20 g of xylitol * ground into powder (or 25 g of erythritol * ground into powder)

With ice cream

450ml 3.5% milk or coconut milk (vegan version)

210 g cream N.B. vegan

150 g of powdered erythritol *

120 g of xylitol * ground into powder

3 g of xanthan gum * or guar or 1.5 g of locust bean gum

3 inulin * or vodka

Vanilla extract * to taste

80 g of frozen, thawed or fresh strawberries

20 g of cocoa powder * without oil

To decorate

fresh berries and finely grated low-carb chocolate to taste

PREPARATION

For the base, melt the low-carb chocolate with the hazelnut butter and xylitol.

Add the chopped hazelnuts and spread them in a removable pan (about 18 cm) with parchment paper and press well.

Put the bottom in the freezer for about 30 minutes. In the meantime, you can prepare the ice cream paste.

For the ice cream mixture, first mix all the dry ingredients (except cocoa powder) and then mix everything with the milk. If you use vodka instead of inulin, you need to add it now as well.

Whip the cream until thick and incorporate it.

Divide the ice cream dough into about three equal portions.

Spread the first portion on the floor and freeze for about 2 hours.

Mix the second portion with the cocoa powder and spread it over the first layer once frozen. The ice cream cake took about 2 hours.

Mash the strawberries, mix with the third portion and roll out the second layer. Freeze the ice cream cake again for about 2 hours.

Before serving, the ice cream cake can be decorated as desired, for example with berries of your choice and grated low-carb chocolate.

About 10 minutes before cutting, the ice cream cake should be removed from the freezer and then cut, preferably with a large knife previously heated in hot water.

10
SUGAR-FREE ICE CREAM: THE BASIC RECIPE

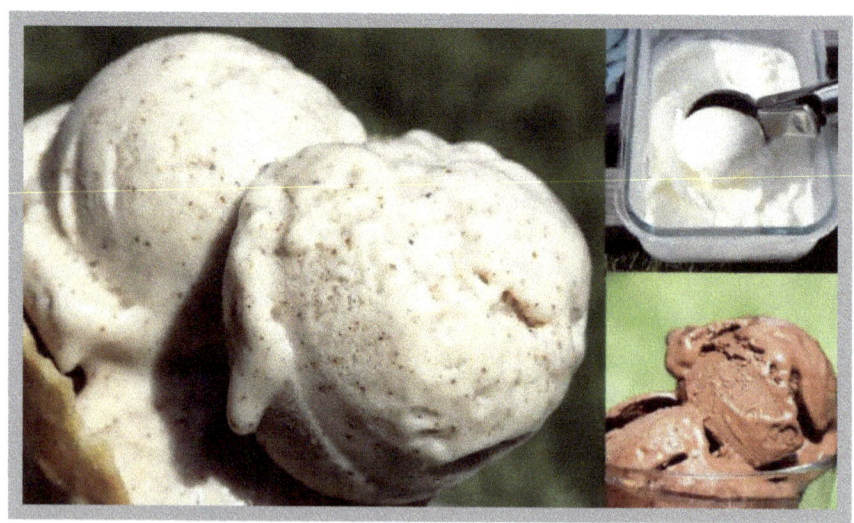

5 MINUTES.

INGREDIENTS

50 g of powdered erythritol *
40 g of xylitol * ground into powder
1 g of xanthan gum * or guar or 1.5 g of locust bean gum
150ml vegan coconut milk, alternatively milk (3.5%)
70 g cream n.B. vegan
1 inulin * or vodka
Vanilla extract * to taste

PREPARATION

PREPARATION with the ice cream maker
   Mix all the dry ingredients.
   start by Attach the wet ingredients and mix everything until smooth with a stir stick.
   Freeze the ice in the refrigerator.
   Preparation without machine for ice cream
   Mix all the dry ingredients, then mix everything with the milk.
   Whip the cream until thick and incorporate it.
   Freeze the ice cream mass and, if possible, stir every 30-60 minutes so that as few ice crystals as possible are formed.

⓫ WATER ICE WITHOUT SUGAR

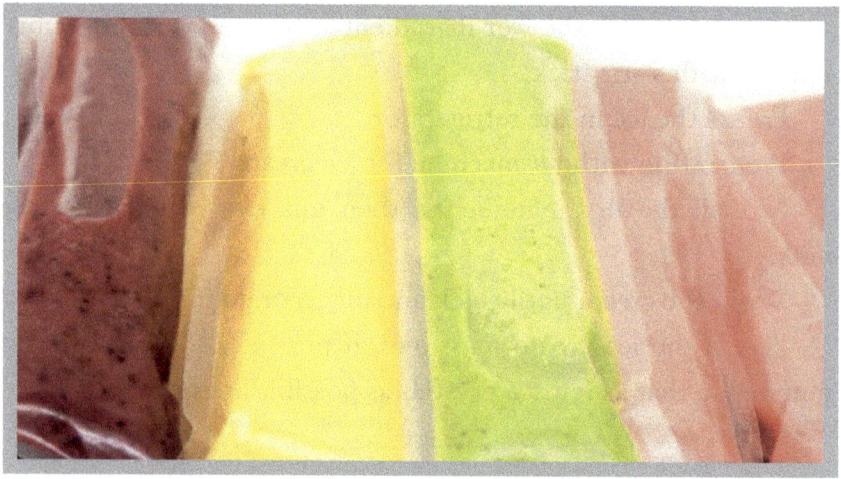

10 MINUTES.

INGREDIENTS
Yellow water ice

150 g papaya
150 g frozen mango
150 g of yogurt 10%
100 ml of water
Frozen green water
Approx. 4 kiwis 250 gr
200 ml of water
50 g fresh baby spinach
30 g almond butter
Purple icy water
200 g frozen blueberries
150 g of yogurt 10%
100 ml of water
1 teaspoon Ceylon cinnamon *
Pink water ice
300 g of yogurt 10%
150 g frozen raspberries
150 g of fresh strawberries

PREPARATION

For the different types of ice cream, it is enough to combine all the ingredients in a blender and mix them finely.

Pour the mixtures into popsicle molds, ideally with a funnel, and freeze overnight.

⑫ ICED COFFEE WITHOUT SUGAR

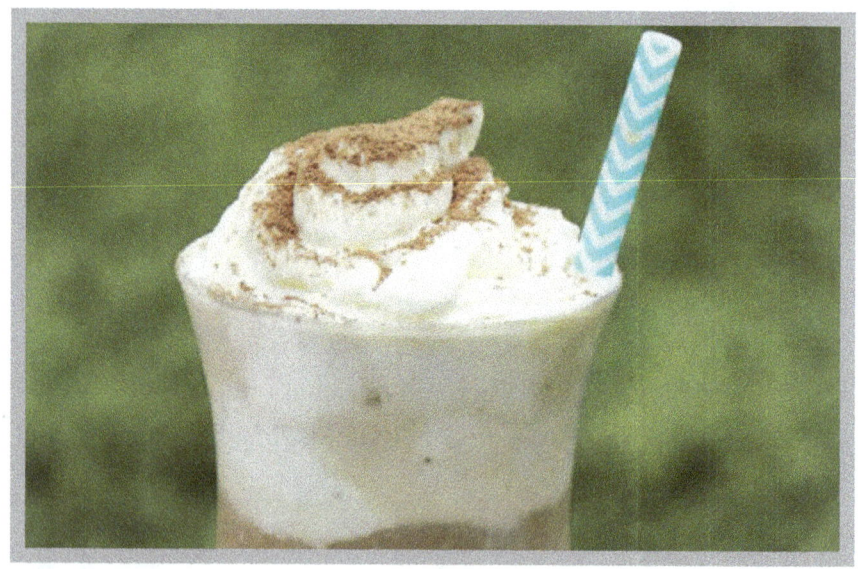

5 minutes.

. . .

INGREDIENTS

200 ml of cold coffee

50 ml of almond milk *

5 ice cubes

2 scoops of sugar-free vanilla ice cream

Decorate

50 g of whipped cream

Cocoa powder * to taste

PREPARATION

Put the ice cubes in a large glass.

Add the cold coffee, almond milk, and 2 scoops of vanilla ice cream.

Finally, the iced coffee can be decorated with whipped cream and cocoa powder.

Have fun now!

13
3 INGREDIENTS SKYR SUGAR FREE ICE CREAM

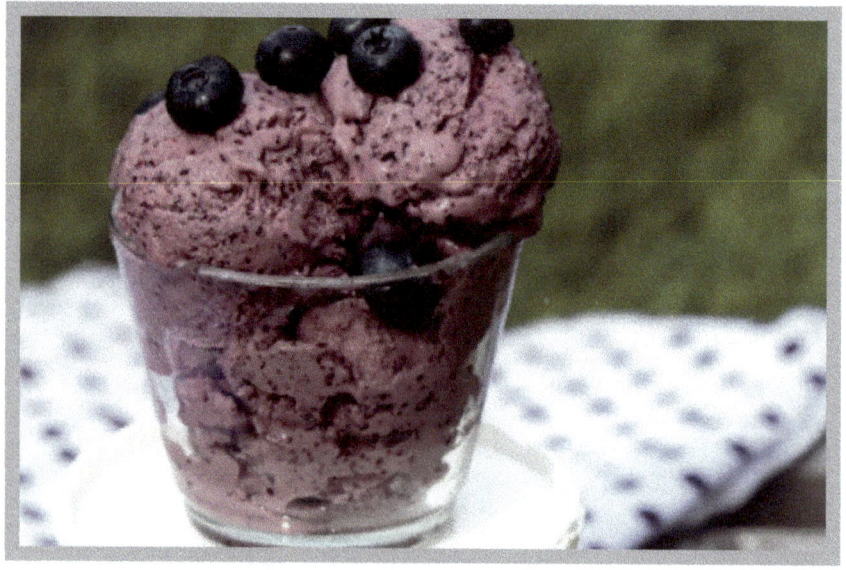

5 MINUTES.

. . .

INGREDIENTS

150 ml of coconut drink *
70 g of cream n.B. vegan
50 g of erythritol powder *
40 g of xylitol * alternatively in Vita fiber powder
25 g of dry coconut *
0.5 g guar gum *
0.5 g xanthan gum *
1 tablespoon of inulin for a little more creaminess

PREPARATION

Preparation with the ice cream machine

Mix all dry ingredients.

Add the wet ingredients and mix everything gently with a stick.

Freeze the ice in the fridge.

Preparation without ice cream machine

Mix all the dry ingredients together, then mix everything with the coconut drink and dried coconut.

Beat the cream until stiff and work.

Freeze the ice cream batter and stir every 30-60 minutes so that as few ice crystals as possible form.

15
UNSWEETENED ICE CREAM POWDER FOR MILK ICE CREAM

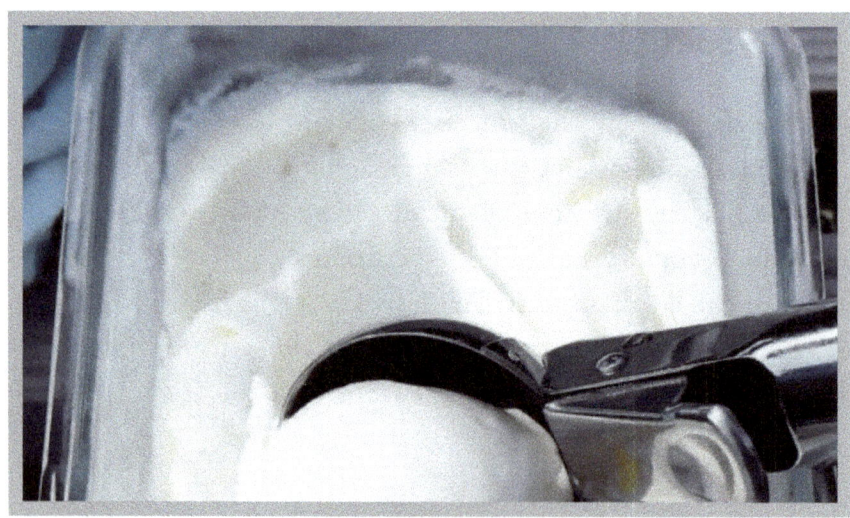

5 minutes.

INGREDIENTS

For ice cream powder

50 g of erythritol powder *

40 g of xylitol * alternatively in Vita fiber powder

1 g xanthan gum * or guar gum or 1.5 g locust bean gum

1 tablespoon inulin * for extra creaminess

equally

150 ml of 3.5% milk or coconut milk (vegan version)

70 g of cream n.B. vegan

PREPARATION

For ice cream, simply mix all the ingredients in a bowl and pour into a sealable container until ready to use.

Making ice cream with the fridge

Mix the powdered ice, milk and cream well with a whisk and then fill the refrigerator.

Making ice cream without an ice machine

Mix the powdered ice and milk well with a whisk.

try Beat the cream until stiff and then add it to the ice cream and milk mixture.

Pour the ice cream batter into a freezer-safe container and freeze.

Stir the ice approximately every 30-60 minutes as it freezes so that as few ice crystals form as possible.

LOW CARB LEMON ICE CREAM WITH BASIL

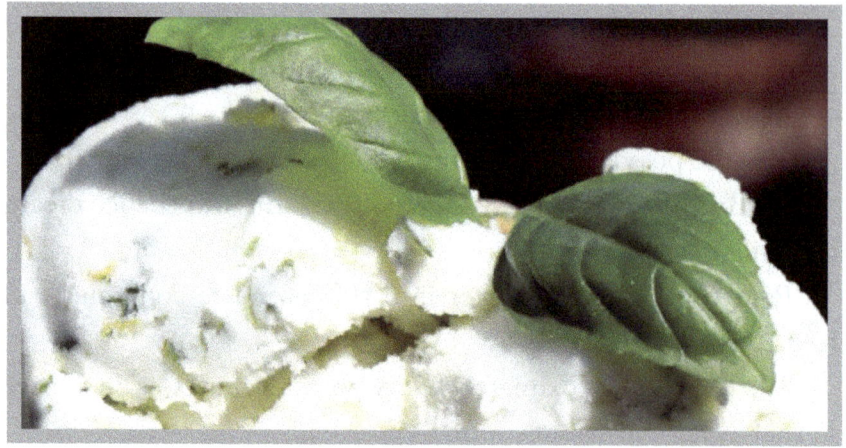

5 MINUTES.

INGREDIENTS

150ml 3.5% milk or coconut milk (vegan version)

70 g cream n.B. vegan

50 g of powdered erythritol *

40 g of xylitol * alternatively powdered Vita fiber

0.5 g of guar gum *
0.5 g xanthan gum *
1 lemon
1 inulin * for extra creaminess
Finely chopped leaves of 2 basil stalks

PREPARATION

Grate the lemon peel finely and squeeze half a lemon's juice.

Using the ice cream machine to make the ice cream

Combine all dry ingredients in a large mixing bowl.

With a stir stick, combine the wet ingredients and stir until smooth.

In the refrigerator, freeze the ice.

Ice cream preparation without the use of a gadget

Combine dry ingredients in a mixing bowl, then add the milk, lemon juice, lemon zest, and basil.

Whip the cream till it reaches the desired consistency, then fold it in.

Freeze the ice cream mass and stir it every 30-60 minutes to avoid forming ice crystals.

17
LOW CARB ALMOND ICE CREAM

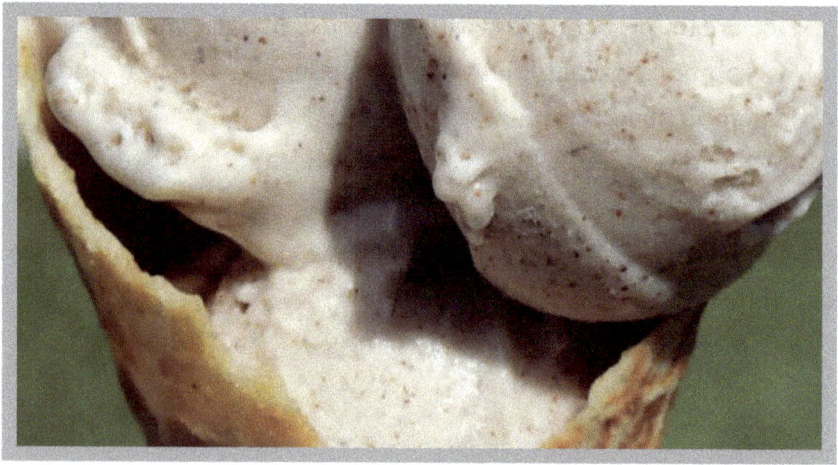

5 minutes.

INGREDIENTS
   150ml 3.5% milk or coconut milk (vegan version)

70 g cream n.B. vegan

60 g of almond butter

50 g of powdered erythritol *

40 g of xylitol * alternatively powdered Vita fiber

0.5 g of guar gum *

0.5 g xanthan gum *

1 inulin * for extra creaminess

PREPARATION

Preparation with the ice cream maker

Mix all the dry ingredients.

With a stir stick, combine the wet ingredients and stir until smooth.

Freeze the ice in the refrigerator.

Preparation without machine for ice cream

Inside a big mixing bowl, combine all of the dry ingredients, then add the milk and almond butter.

Whip the cream until it is thick and fluffy, then fold it in.

Freeze the ice cream mass and stir it every 30-60 minutes to ensure that no ice crystals form.

18
LOW CARB CARAMEL ICE CREAM

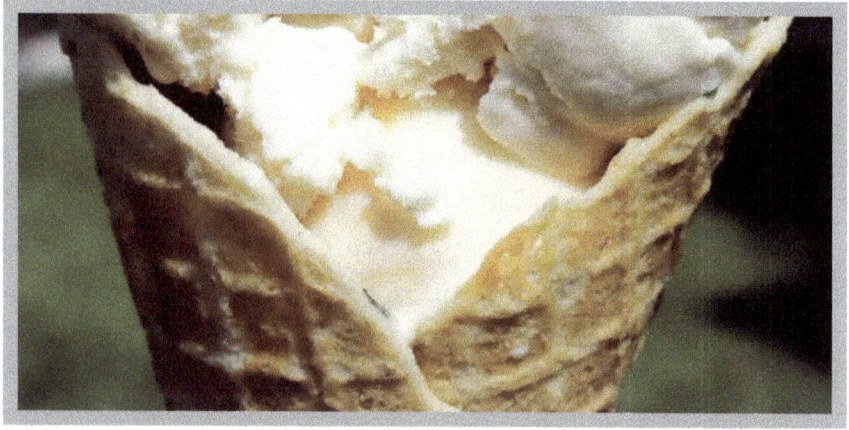

20 MINUTES.

INGREDIENTS
  50 g of powdered erythritol *
  40 g of xylitol * ground into powder

0.5 g of guar gum *
0.5 g xanthan gum *
150ml 3.5% milk or coconut milk (vegan version)
70 g cream n.B. vegan
1 inulin * or vodka
1/2 serving of sugar-free caramel

PREPARATION

Preparation with the ice cream maker
Blend erythritol, xylitol, xanthan gum, guar gum, and inulin.
Add the milk and cream and mix everything until smooth.
Pour the mixture into the refrigerator and let it freeze.
Pour the ice cream into a freezer container, add the caramel (preferably cooled to room temperature) and fold it with a few turns of your hand.
Freeze the ice cream for at least another 60 minutes before consuming it.
Preparation without machine for ice cream
Blend erythritol, xylitol, xanthan gum, guar gum, and inulin.
Add the milk and mix everything together until smooth.
Whip the cream until thick and incorporate it.
Put the ice cream in a freezer container, add the caramel and fold it with a few turns of your hand.
Freeze the ice cream mass and, if possible, stir every 30-60 minutes so that as few ice crystals as possible are formed.

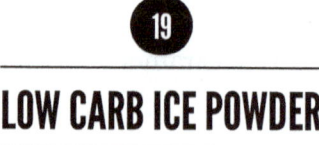

LOW CARB ICE POWDER

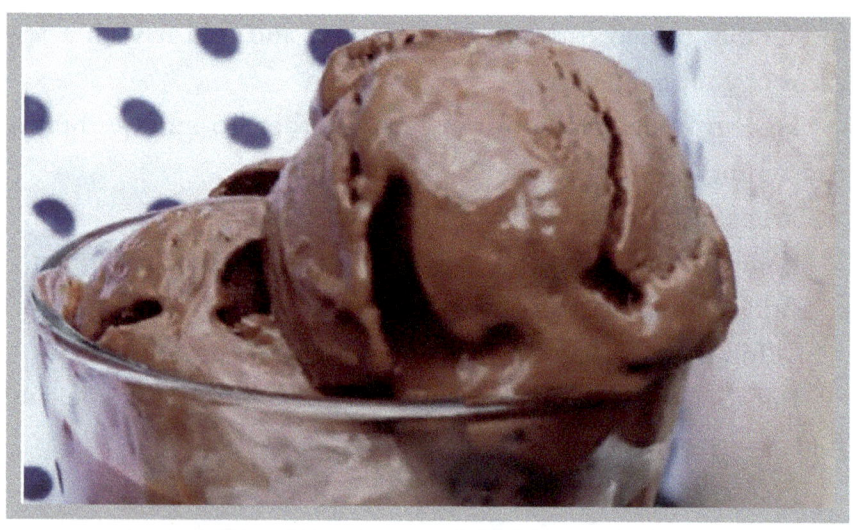

5 minutes.

INGREDIENTS

For the powdered ice cream
20 g of cocoa powder * without oil
50 g of powdered erythritol *
40 g of xylitol * alternatively powdered Vita fiber
1 g of xanthan gum * or guar or 1.5 g of locust bean gum
1 inulin * for extra creaminess
What's more
150ml 3.5% milk or coconut milk (vegan version)
70 g cream n.B. vegan

PREPARATION

For ice cream, simply mix all the ingredients in a bowl and pour them into a sealable container until you are ready to use it.

Making ice cream with the ice cream maker.

Mix the powdered ice, milk and cream well with a whisk and then fill the refrigerator.

Making ice cream without an ice machine

Mix the powdered ice and milk well with a whisk.

Whip the cream until stiff, then add it to the ice cream and milk mixture.

Pour the ice cream dough into a freezer-safe container and freeze it.

Stir the ice every 30 to 60 minutes as it freezes so that as few ice crystals form as possible.

20
LOW CARB NOUGAT ICE CREAM

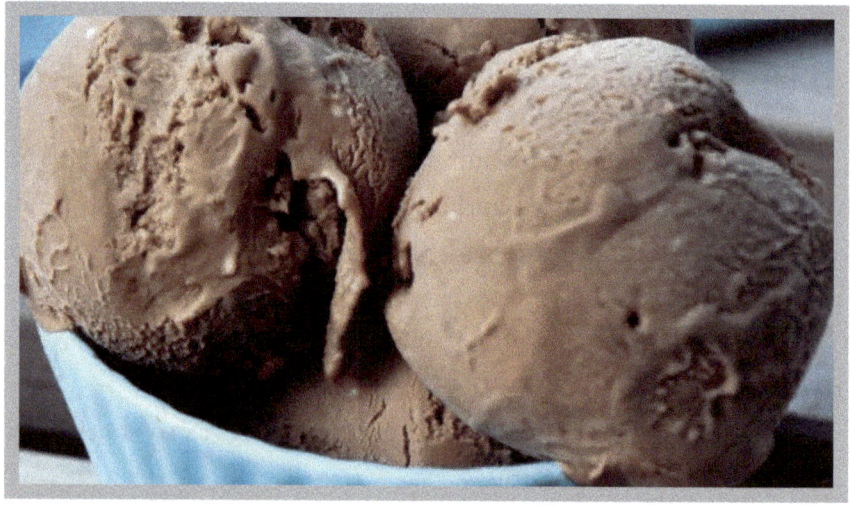

10 MINUTES.

INGREDIENTS
150 ml of milk or coconut milk

70 ml heavy cream

60 g unsweetened hazelnut nougat cream

30 g of erythritol powder *

20 g xylitol * ground into powder

1 g xanthan gum * or guar gum or 1.5 g locust bean gum

1 tablespoon inulin * or vodka

PREPARATION

Preparation with the ice cream machine

Mix all dry ingredients.

Add the wet ingredients and mix everything gently with a stick.

Freeze the ice in the fridge.

Preparation without ice cream machine. Mix all the dry ingredients, then mix everything with the milk.

Beat the cream until stiff and work.

Freeze the ice cream batter and, if possible, stir every 30-60 minutes so that as few ice crystals form as possible.

LOW CARB CUCUMBER ICE CREAM

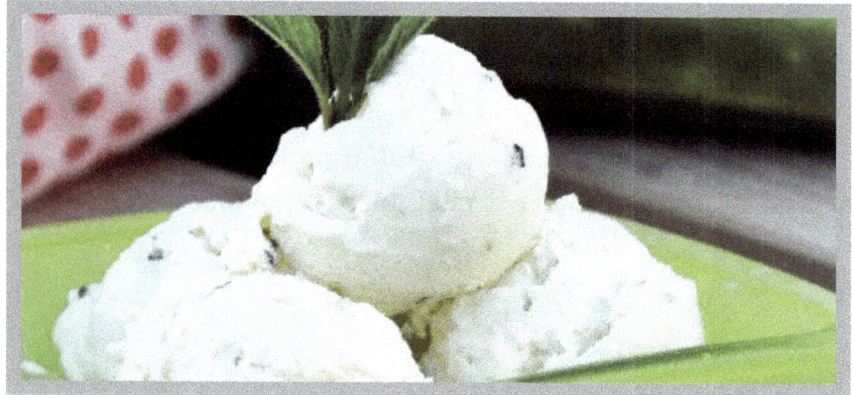

10 MINUTES.

INGREDIENTS

1/2 snake cucumber smoothie

50 g of erythritol powder *

40 g xylitol * ground into powder

1 g xanthan gum * or guar gum or 1.5 g locust bean gum

100 ml of milk or coconut milk (vegan version)

70 ml of cream n.B. vegan

1 tablespoon inulin * or vodka

10 minced mint leaves

PREPARATION

Preparation with the ice cream machine

Mix all dry ingredients.

Add the wet ingredients and mix everything gently with a stick.

Freeze the ice in the fridge.

Preparation without ice cream machine

Mix all the dry ingredients, then mix everything with the milk.

Beat the cream until stiff and work.

Freeze the ice cream batter and, if possible, stir every 30-60 minutes so that as few ice crystals form as possible.

22

LOW CARB ICE MIRACLE

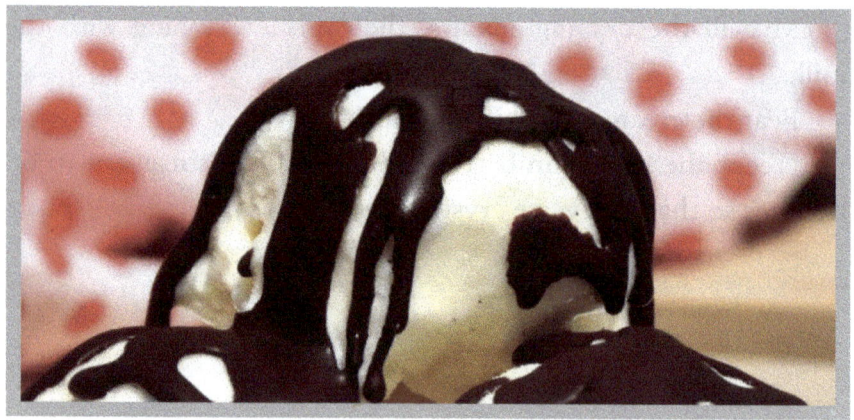

3 MINUTES.

INGREDIENTS
  60 g of cocoa mass *
  20 g coconut oil *

If you don't like it so bitter, you can add a little powdered erythritol if needed.

PREPARATION

Melt the cocoa mass and coconut oil together.

Those who prefer a "sweeter" taste may want to add a little powdered erythritol.

Let the chocolate sauce cool to room temperature and pour it over ice if necessary. Now you can see how it forms a hard chocolate crust on your ice cream.

MAKE YOURSELF LOW CARB ICE CREAM - ICE CREAM RECIPES

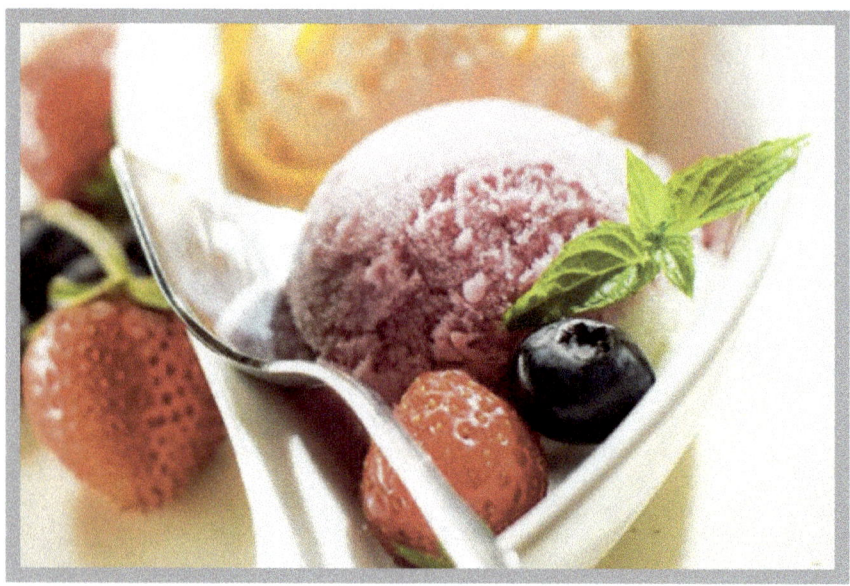

30 MINUTES

INGREDIENTS

500 g of frozen berries

100-150 g of xylitol (xucker)

100ml of cream (you can also use milk)

2 drops of vanilla flavor

PREPARATION

Put the frozen berries in a blender along with the xucker. Gradually pour in the cream during the mixing process until the mixture is thick and creamy. Season your low carb ice cream with vanilla and enjoy it right away.

TIP: you can also freeze the dough. Allow to defrost briefly before serving.

OTHER LOW CARB ice cream recipes:

24
MAKE YOURSELF LOW CARB RASPBERRY ICE CREAM

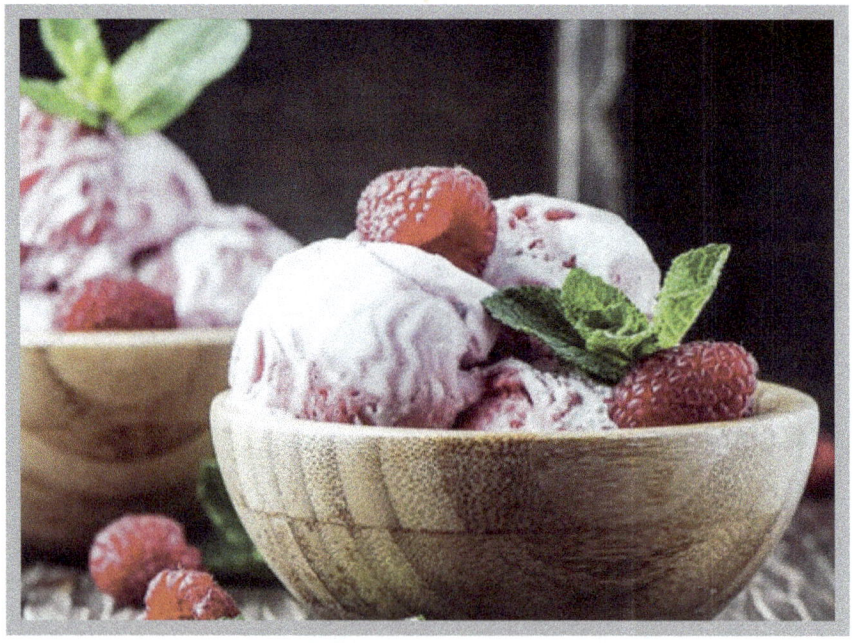

5 MINUTES.

. . .

INGREDIENTS

400 g of frozen raspberries

80 g of powdered sugar

200 g of yogurt

100 ml of whipped cream

PREPARATION

Put the frozen raspberries, the xucker powder, the yogurt and the cream in a blender. Stir vigorously and voila, your low carb yogurt and raspberry ice cream is ready.

TIP: You can also freeze the leftovers and thaw them briefly before serving.

㉕
LOW CARB STRAWBERRY YOGURT POPSICLES

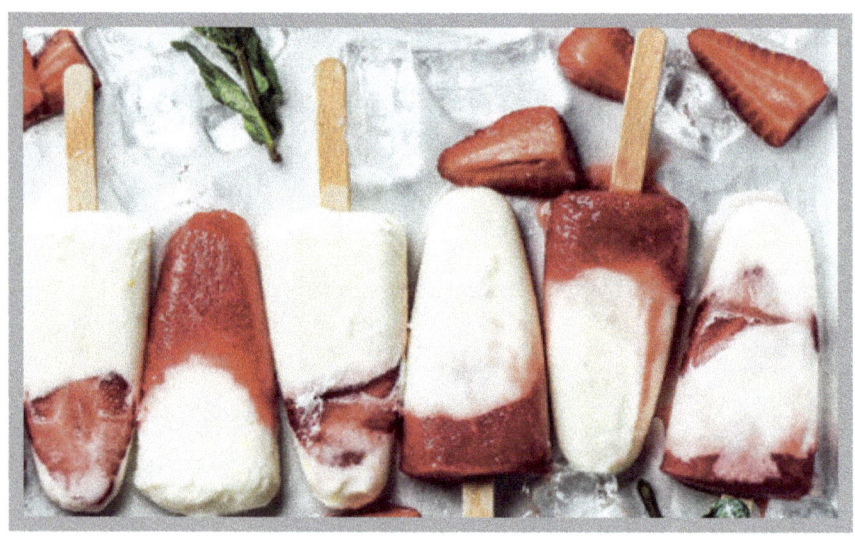

20 MINUTES

INGREDIENTS

200 grams of fresh or frozen strawberries

200 grams of yogurt

3 tablespoons xylitol

xucker

Vanilla pulp half pod

2 tablespoons of cream or coconut milk

PREPARATION

Mash the strawberries with half of the xucker. Mix the yogurt with the rest of the xucker, the cream or coconut milk and the pulp of the vanilla bean.

First, pour the fruit mixture into two molds and the yogurt mixture into two molds and cover them with the other mixture. Insert the popsicles and freeze them for at least 4 hours.

Tip: Ice can be easily removed from the mold if it is briefly held under running water.

26
LOW CARB BLUEBERRY CREAMY RICE

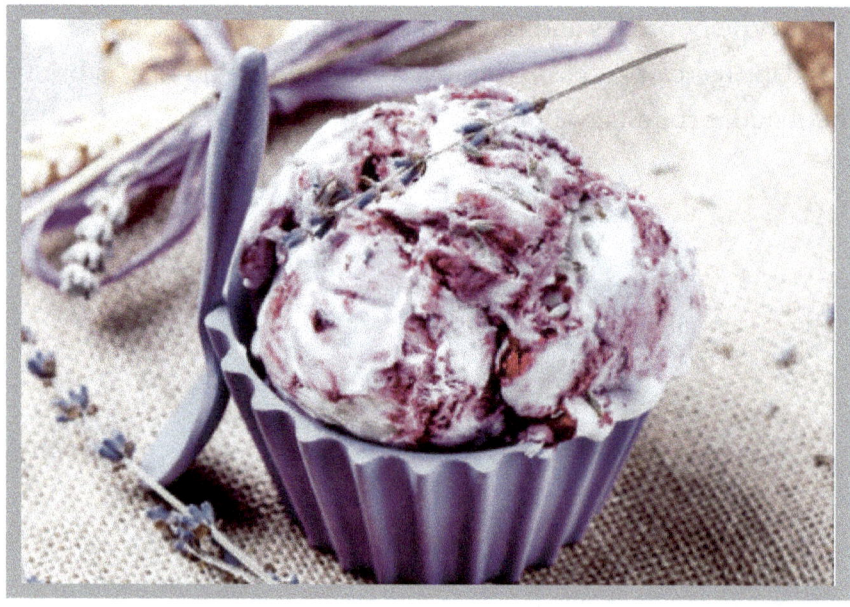

15 MINUTES

. . .

INGREDIENTS

200 grams of blueberries
4 tablespoons xylitol xucker
Organic half lemon juice
2 egg yolks
1 whole egg
300 ml of cream

PREPARATION

Coarsely blend the blueberries with the lemon juice and half of the xucker. Mix the egg and yolks with the rest of the xucker until fluffy. Whip the cream until stiff and then mix with the quantity of egg.

Pour into a mold and coarsely add the fruit puree so that the fruit and cream do not mix completely and create a beautiful pattern. This works best with a wooden spoon.

It is best to freeze ice overnight, but for at least 8 hours. Shape a scoop of ice cream into beautiful balls and place them in muffin bowls.

Low-carb ice cream can be garnished with fresh berries. Of course, instead of blueberries, you can also use currants, strawberries or raspberries.

27

LOW CARB BLUEBERRY YOGURT

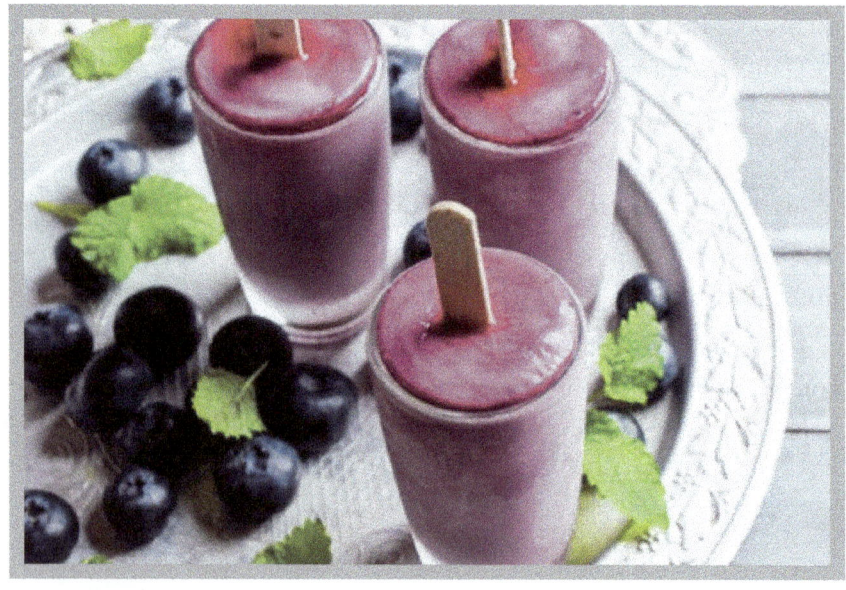

INGREDIENTS

   350 grams of blueberries

   300 grams of yogurt

4 tablespoons of xylitol

xucker

2 tablespoons of quark cream cheese

PREPARATION

Mix the blueberries with a hand mixer and pass them through a sieve. Mix the yogurt with the xucker and the quark cream until you get a homogeneous mixture with the fruit.

Pour into glasses and dip a stem in the mixture. Freeze for at least 5 hours.

Tip: Low-carb ice can be easily removed from the glass by briefly holding it under hot water. Be careful not to wait too long for it to melt in your mouth and not in the glass.

28

LOW CARB RASPBERRY YOGURT CREAMY ICE CREAM

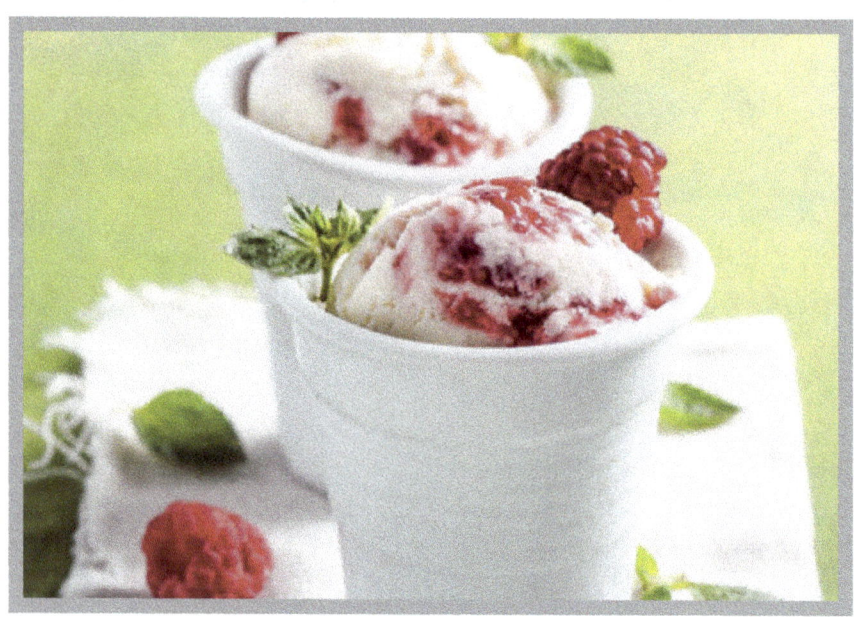

INGREDIENTS

200 grams of fresh or frozen raspberries

4 tablespoons xylitol Xucker
2 egg yolks
1 whole egg
100 ml of yogurt
100 ml of cream

PREPARATION

Mash the raspberries with a fork. Beat half of the xucker with the yolk and whole egg until fluffy. Whip the cream with the rest of the xucker. Add the yogurt to the egg mixture. Carefully incorporate the cream and mix with the fruit. Freeze everything for at least 8 hours.

Cut out nice balls with an ice cream scoop or measuring cup and serve.

Tip: if you like it particularly fresh, you can mash the raspberries with a few mint leaves and add the juice of half an organic lime.

29

LOW CARB CREAMY RASPBERRY ICE CREAM

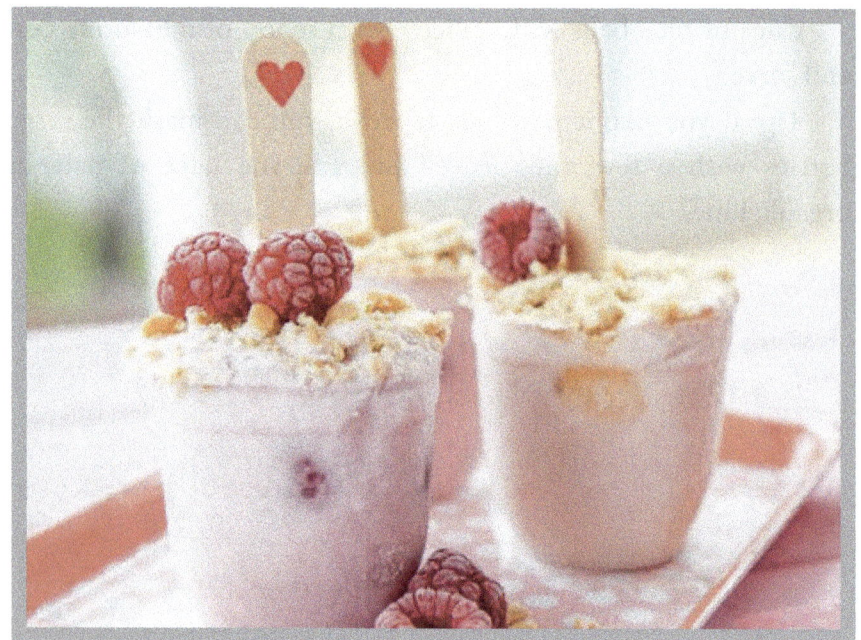

INGREDIENTS
160 grams of raspberries

80 grams of low carb cookies
150 ml of cream
300 grams of quark cream
4 tablespoons xylitol
xucker
Organic lime juice

PREPARATION

Mash the fruit with a fork. Set aside some fruit for garnish. Crumble the cookies. Set 2 tablespoons of crumbs aside for garnish. Whip the cream until stiff peaks.

Mix the curd with the fruit, xucker, biscuits and lime juice until smooth and carefully pour in the cream.

Pour the mixture into the glasses and sprinkle with the remaining biscuits.

Freeze now for at least 6 hours, but preferably overnight. Garnish with fruit before serving.

The cookies in the ice cream create a special crunch and make this ice cream a very special pleasure experience.

www.ingramcontent.com/pod-product-compliance
Lightning Source LLC
Chambersburg PA
CBHW071126030426
42336CB00013BA/2211